I0439428

51 motivational thoughts and quotes that will change the way you think as an athlete forever

Written By Dr. Sourr

ISBN-13: 978-1494719746
ISBN-10: 1494719746

Dedicated to all the athletes who have risked everything to capture a dream that only they can see come true

1#
[No matter how rough it may seem keep believing in your dream and believe it is possible to achieve your dream, you must have faith.]

2#
[Faith is like a seed of that vision that only you can see happen it will truly grow when you nurture and take care of it everyday.]

3#
[Faith is knowing you can still win even after you've made huge mistakes at the start.]

4#
[Once you lose faith in yourself and stop believing you've just lost the greatest opportunity to make your vision or dream become a reality at that very moment you stopped believing.]

5#

[Everyone thought Albert Einstein was a lunatic because of his ideas so don't let anyone around you think your idea or dream is insane as well, believe in your vision and dream no one can see what you can see but you.]

6#
[All things are possible to those who believe.]

7#
[The impossible is possible by believing and having faith that the impossible is possible.]

8#
[Know that you were born to do what you believe in.]

9#
[Know that you have a chance to make history every time you compete.]

10#
[Know that you are born for greatness.]

11#

[Your that new athlete! Your that new greatness! Your that new historical story that the new generation of people will talk about and read stories about. The people who you looked up to and who you thought were a great inspiration to you are either dead or retired, YOU ARE THAT NEW ATHLETE!]

12#
[You are that new athlete that everyone dreams and hopes to see, the old athletes have either died or become boring you are the new upcoming athlete of this generation that has now arrived.]

13#
[Become your dream and make it a reality don't settle to become an ordinary athlete. People do want and dream about seeing an extraordinary athlete that has skills beyond its time.]

14#
[What ever you dream about accomplishing you have already made it possible to accomplish just by visualizing it itself.]

15#
[What ever you dream about doing already exists, it will eventually come true only if you have the will power to commit to it and turn it into a reality.]

16#
[Your dream will come true if you dedicate and sacrifice your life completely to it, it takes time for visions to become a reality, and you will have your time.]

17#

[If you truly want what you dream about becoming, change today at this very moment because tomorrow does not even exist yet, you must put in work to become what you want today because that's who you are truly capable of becoming.]

18#

[Some athletes say "I'm going to train tomorrow or I'm going to train harder next month" but the truth is tomorrow does not even exist yet you have a chance and the power to change the future today not tomorrow.]

19#
[Stats are just numbers recorded from the past.]

20#

[What ever you do today becomes part of your past, time never stops for anyone and the future does not exist yet. You can still change your future today, you are in control of whatever situation you are in.]

21#

[The future does not exist yet stop thinking about it, don't let time pass you by and don't be a spectator, be involved with the present moment which is today and make it a goal to get better at your craft every single day even if its only for thirty minutes.]

22#

[There is not a future yet, there is only the present moment which is now, you can change the present moment by putting in action! Not speaking, not dreaming, and not waiting for an opportunity. Actions speak louder than words, if you want something work for it and go for it, don't be afraid to fail.]

23#

[Just SHOW UP, you will not become what you want to become by hoping on a miracle or dramatic event to happen. If you don't show up in life things most likely will not change. For example, you will not win the lottery by waiting at home and hoping, you must SHOW UP to the store and buy a ticket for a chance to win.]

24#

[It takes time, it takes hard training, it takes commitment, it takes sacrifice, it takes dedication to make a dream come true because there are many others who want to accomplish the same dream as much as you do.]

25#

["your body is your slave!" You tell it what to do, don't give up when your body is in pain, telling you to give up, and telling you to stop training. In your mind tell your body that its your slave when it wants to give up on you.]

26#

[You can either take the pain and soreness from training now and be known as a champion your entire life or you can either give up now and be just another ordinary athlete that tried his best, your in control, and you choose.]

27#
[When your muscles are tremendously sore just smile and be happy because all that pain that you feel will be worth the success and is only a small part of something even greater that you are trying to accomplish.]

28#

[What ever you can do in training you will be able to do in competition so training is always a big and an important part to help you achieve your dream. Don't train a little bit and then expect to win by luck and hope, always remember that there is always someone training and dedicating there life to be the best and better than YOU.]

29#
[Train to become the champ of champs, don't train to become an ordinary champion just
like everyone else, train to become the champs of ALL champs.]

30#
[Train like there's always some one better than you, no matter how good you may think you already are.]

31#
[Make it a goal to become so great that you might even be memorized fifty years from now, be greatness!]

32#
[You must visualize all the out comes in all situations, the bad and the good like visualizing the crowd booing at you or you coming back from a bad loss, visualize all possible outcomes so that your mind will always be ready mentally to handle what could happen in the future.]

33#
[Visualization is practicing an outcome inside your head that could actually happen, visualize your come back from a failure or mistake, visualize what you'll do right after you win or score a goal, visualizing helps you prepare for mistakes and even helps you succeed.]

34#
[Be creative and use visualization as a tool during training and competition. For example, visualize that a magnet is pulling you towards the finish line during a race or when you weight lifting on a bench press visualize a magnet pulling the weights up when you lift the heavy weights up, BE CREATIVE.]

35#

[Always be positive and say positive words and phrases in your head while you train like "I am the best, I am the greatest, no body can beat me or stop me, I will win this competition coming up, my body is my slave it listens to me I don't give up!"]

36#
[There will be many ups and downs, have faith and keep training if you are already deep into the sport, to reach the top of a mountain the road is not always perfectly strait.]

37#

[Even though people don't see what you are doing behind the scenes don't cheat while you train, make sure that when you train you are always training effectively, all your training will show in competition and people will see that.]

38#
[Don't train to be seen by people or just to look cool, train to be the best, train effectively every single time even when you are not seen by people.]

39#
[All your hard work, training, and dedication will show in competition.]

40#
[Have a purpose because with no purpose you will never have drive to become the greatest.]

41#
[You could be someone that trains the most effectively in the entire world but never make it because you have no real purpose or no real reason to accomplish your dream.]

42#
[When you are feeling down always think of your purpose and the reason why you are trying to accomplish your goal in the first place, ask yourself "why am trying to accomplish this."]

43#
[What is your purpose and your reason for accomplishing your dream? Money and materials will always fade away.]

44#
[Being the greatest means you always push yourself harder and you are always ready to face who ever wants your spot as the greatest.]

45#
[Being the greatest means more than striving to be the best only one time, being the greatest means you are always ready and prepared mentally and physically to compete against any body and always come out on top no matter what the situation may be.]

46#

[Treat every single game, every single competition, every single fight like its the play offs or like its your last game to show that you are the greatest no matter how small the situation may seem to you that way when you really make it to the play offs your mind will already be mentally prepared and ready for it.]

47#
[Once your at the top of your game is when you really have to train and push yourself
even more because people will expect more from you.]

48#
[Never lose faith.]

49#
[Never stop believing.]

50#
[Never stop training, be consistent, and stay committed to accomplishing your goals.]

51#

[To be the greatest you must dedicate your life to be the greatest; you must know that you are the greatest so become the greatest and act like the greatest!]